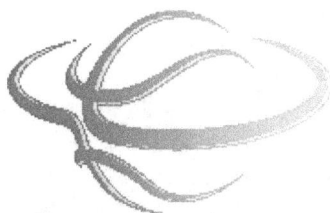

iTeachBasketball.com

BECOME A BETTER BASKETBALL COACH

VOLUME 1

FOCUS ON FUNDAMENTALS
- FITNESS - MOVEMENT -
- BALL HANDLING -

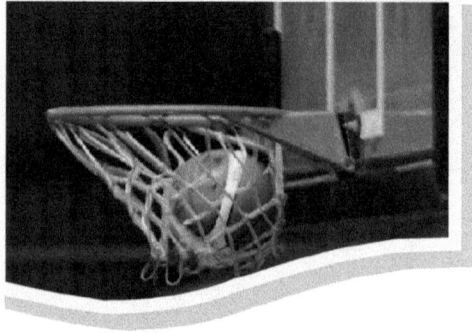

ISBN: 978-0-9875084-0-9

Published by Michael Haynes, trading as iTeachBasketball.com

Copyright © 2013

GET THE FUNDAMENTALS RIGHT

This book will help you develop the fundamentals skills of your athletes and their understanding of the game, which is a key to them enjoying the game. Some activities are designed for a small number of athletes (3 or 4), however you can have your team do a number of activities at the same time.

Some athletes only want to practice shooting and find activities that focus on other fundamental skills "boring". You can avoid boredom by using activities that keep athletes active and are challenging.

Remember, the key to teaching is *NOT* the drills you use – your teaching points and what you emphasise is most important. In this regard your actions speak louder than your words. For example, it doesn't matter how many times you tell the athletes to use a jump stop. If you don't correct them if they don't use a jump stop, you are not teaching them to use the jump stop.

The biggest mistake that coaches make is to focus on the particular "drill" that they are running. They correct the athletes mostly on where to run or what to do next to keep the "drill" going—they are teaching how to do the drill.

But, they don't teach them the fundamental skills and they are not teaching them how to play the game!

Instead, each activity should be to an opportunity for players to practice, refine and develop the skills they are working on, NOT the logistics of a drill!

Don't stop the activity every time you notice something wrong. Instead, coach "on the run" as much as possible. Giving short, specific feedback whilst the activity continues.

When giving feedback, say the player's name first (to get their attention). Preferably be close enough to them so that you don't have to yell. For longer instruction, have the athlete step out of the drill, rather than stopping the whole activity. However, get them back in as quickly as you can!

Use positive language when you are giving feedback - tell them what to do rather than saying "No" or "Don't" continuously. Always acknowledge when they improve or get it right.

When introducing an activity, give the athletes 1 or 2 teaching points and use "key words" to describe them. Once the activity starts take the time to observe as the athletes "explore" the skill.

It is understandable that the team may get some of the "mechanics" of the activity wrong, particularly when they are first doing it.

Rather than stopping the drill:

(a) Encourage the athletes to be vocal and encouraging other team mates in what to do;

(b) Coach "on the run" - stand next to athletes that are struggling and talk to them about what they have to do next;

(c) Don't put an athlete that is unsure about the drill, at the front of the line. Let them see how the activity works first.

During the activity repeat your key words or teaching points to give concise feedback, rather than wordy explanations of what they should have done or what they did wrong.

It is also a good idea at the end of training to give athletes a summary of the key words that you are using - this is also great for parents!

This book includes drills that I have created as well as many drills that I have seen other coaches use or have been fortunate to work with those coaches.

However there is no "magic" in any of the activities you will find in this book - the magic comes from you and your focus on teaching the fundamentals!

Good luck with your coaching.

Coach Haynes

What's inside?

The Coach's Classroom

A coach is a teacher, the court is their classroom and athletes are their students.

The coach's success depends upon their ability to inspire, motivate and guide the athletes to grasp the fundamental building blocks that will help them solve any problem that they come across.

To learn, athletes need to be given the chance to get things wrong, to explore how to do it and to understand why it is done that way. When they understand "why", they will be able to apply the knowledge to a range of situations, not just the context in which the originally learnt the skill.

When first teaching a skill, give players the chance to rehearse it without worrying about opposition players, the position of their teammates etc. Only use this "closed" style of learning for a short time!

Players need to develop the ability to play and to do the skills under "game pressure", which means you need to give them the chance to practice using contested activities.

You can make activities contested a number of ways:

- Keeping a "score" and having the players aim to improve their score each time;
- Keeping "score" and comparing that score with other players, again looking for improvement;
- Playing with modified rules against opponents;
- Playing "small sided" games, such as 1v1, 2v1, 2v2, 3v2 etc

The "art of coaching" is your ability to vary the activities that you use in order to emphasise particular concepts or skills. You don't need a lot of different activities but you do need to be well prepared and enthusiastic. Visit our website to see "The Only 10 Drills You need to Coach".

Some tips on varying your activities:

- Restrict the number of dribbles (even to none), to emphasise passing;
- Change how a team scores to emphasise teamwork (eg. by passing the ball to someone in the key);
- Don't let players take the ball out of someone's hands, to emphasise defensive positioning and anticipation in order to steal passes;
- Have uneven numbers on teams, to emphasise the importance of working as a team;
- Make players use their "off" hand, to emphasise the ability to do skills with both hands;
- Restrict roles of some people in the activity (eg they can only pass) to emphasise that scoring is not the only valuable thing you can do (give everyone a turn at being restricted);
- Add "traffic" to your drills by having more than one group on the court at the one time (eg in a full court lay-up drill). This emphasises being aware of where other players are on the court.

Finally, as much as you possibly can "coach on the run". Don't stop activities to give instruction. Instead use concise teaching points (eg "high release" for shooting) to give feedback during the activity.

For your teaching points to be effective, you need to have explained them. You should do this when you first introduce the skill. However, resist the temptation to tell them everything you know about the skill. They wont remember more than one or two things, and you will just confuse them if you tell them "all you know". When planning practice jot down the one or two things that are most important.

It is also a very good idea to give your athletes "homework" sheets, that explain your teaching points. This can be very effective with younger athletes as a guide for their parents. You can also give them some games that they can play at home to practice.

You can get a complete set of homework sheets from our website, www.iTeachBasketball.com

Homework sheets don't have to be complicated. For example, the teaching point "elbow above your eyes" or "high release" is often used with shooting.

Your homework sheet could go into detail about why a high release is important (a higher trajectory has a higher probability of going in) or it could simply have a picture showing an example of what a good shot release looks like.

Here is an example of a homework sheet for shooting:

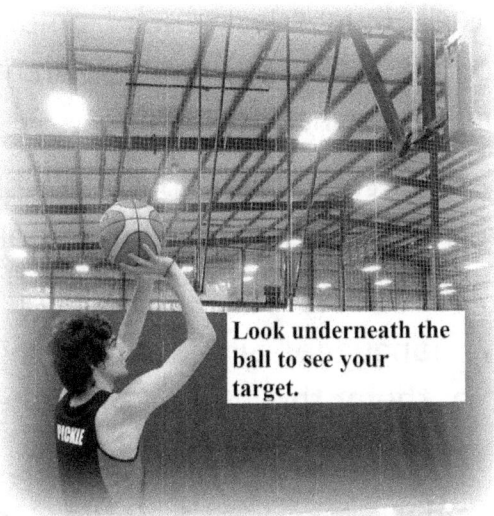

Look underneath the ball to see your target.

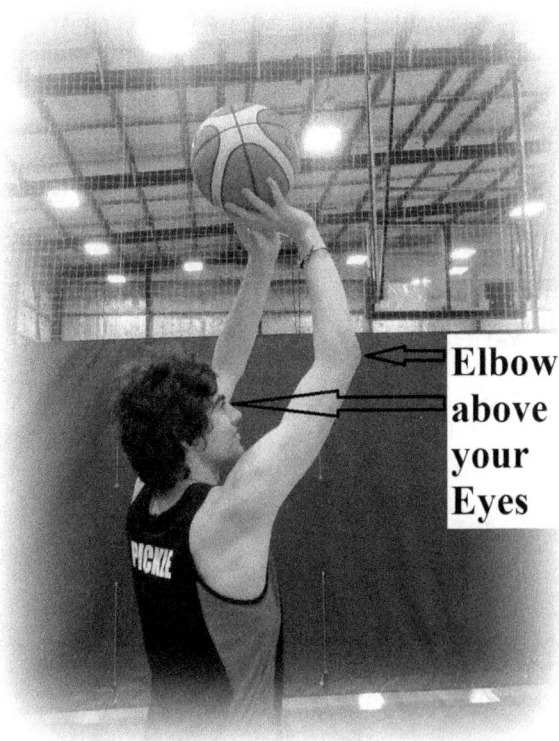

Elbow above your Eyes

Focus on doing

You should use "action oriented" language, which simply means it is more effective to tell athletes what you want them to do, rather than telling them what not to do.

For example, in a dribbling activity saying "look up" or "see me" will be more effective than saying "don't look down".

You should always use positive language, aimed at getting them to do something. Give them the "cure" not the "disease".

Finally, and perhaps most importantly, don't forget to emphasise when an athlete is doing something right! You may particularly need to focus on the "process" rather than the "outcomes".

For example, if you have been teaching a player how to have a good high release when they shoot, they will tend to evaluate whether a shot is good or bad by whether it went in. When they display the high release you've been teaching - praise that and give them the confidence that if they continue to do that they will shoot a higher %.

Sample Training Structure

There is not enough time available to teach all that you know, therefore you must be selective and convey to your players what are the most important parts that they should know.

Tex Winter

In putting together your training session make sure each activity has a purpose, such as:

- Athletic Improvement (developing balance, agility, co-ordination);

- Skill Acquisition (learning, refining or correcting a basketball skill);

- Conditioning (improving aerobic fitness or muscular endurance);

- Game Pressure (executing skills under "game like" pressure).

Many of the activities that you will use will have more than one purpose, however being clear on the main purpose of each activity helps you to include it at the right time in the session.

Activities that focus on athletic improvement or skill acquisition, for example, are best done early in the session, when the athlete's are "fresh".

It is better to have several short breaks rather than one longer break. During breaks, activities such as free throw shooting (or "concept" shooting to practice technique) can be very worthwhile.

At the start of each activity, tell the athletes the main teaching points. Be brief! A good guide when giving feedback or instruction is stick to one minute - after all that's all you have in a time-out!

Teaching points must focus on what players need to learn. Too many coaches teach how the activity runs (eg X shoots, goes over here, dribbles etc) but don't spend sufficient time on their teaching points.

When athletes need correction (and they will), try to identify the "illness", not just the symptom. For example, an athlete may shoot the ball to the left, which could be caused by:

a)   position of their feet;

b)   position of their elbow;

c)   turning their upper body; or

d)   their wrist turning as they shoot the ball.

You would correct each problem differently, so take the time to identify what needs to be corrected.

It is very important that you give the athlete a solution (ie what they need to do) rather than just telling them what they are doing wrong.

For example, if a player shoots the ball "flat", many coaches tell them "don't shoot flat, give the ball air". Does this help the athlete? Give the ball air - do you want them to pump it up?

What the player needs to be taught is how to avoid shooting "flat" and the key to this is pushing up, not out.

The teaching point "elbow higher than your eye" emphasises how to shoot. It gives them a solution - push the ball "up" not "out"

In a one hour training session you could spend time :

Body Movement   **5 mins**
Work on footwork, agility and co-ordination

Ball Handling   **10 mins**
General ball handling and dribbling skills

Passing   **5 mins**
Many activities include passing and you should always insist on good technique. This is an opportunity to introduce your teaching points.

Shooting   **25 mins**
This should include offensive rebounding.

Defence   **15 mins**
This should include defensive rebounding.

Now, you may be thinking "but what about warming up and stretching?". These are important, but don't "waste" your precious training time on them!

Athletes can do their warm up/down or stretching off the court, so that when your session starts they are ready to go. Consider scheduling your session to start 15 minutes before you start on court, to make sure they have time to warm up.

It is also a good idea if athletes have a "yoga mat" to sit on when they are stretching. The floor in a basketball stadium is usually quite cold and sitting down to stretch is counter productive - we want them to "warm up".

You should plan each training session, to make sure you, and the players, get the most out of it. You can get a series of training plans from our website - www.iTeachBasketball.com.

Below is an example format you can use. The pictures of courts at the bottom are for your notes.

Example Session Plan Format

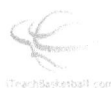

DATE: _____

AIMS OF SESSION:
1. [Briefly, what are you focussing this session]
2. [May be individual skills eg shooting, passing]
3. [May be team skills eg "split line" defence]

EQUIPMENT: [LIST THE EQUIPMENT THAT YOU HAVE/NEED FOR TRAINING]

Time	Drill	Teaching Points	Match Ups
	[Name of Activity]	[2 or 3 teaching points at the most]	[Think about who you want in each group]

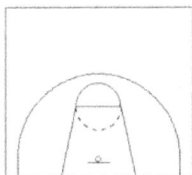

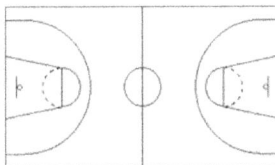

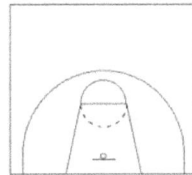

What to Teach?

> *When you step on the floor know **WHAT** you are going to teach, **HOW** you are going to teach it and **WHY** you are going to teach it.*
>
> ### *Tex Winter*

A skills matrix is included on our website, www.iTeachBasketball.com, which gives a guide to when particular skills or concepts should be taught. If you coach juniors, they will all be at different stages of physical and basketball development.

However, all athletes need to be able to:

Moving and Stopping	
Jump Stop:	A jump stop is landing on two feet at the same time. If they have the ball they can choose either foot to pivot. It is good to use when catching a pass and preparing to shoot quickly. Players may overbalance using a jump stop. Avoid this by keeping "nose behind the toes". Jumping higher, which is effective jumping into the key, can help.
Stride Stop:	One foot lands and then the other foot lands. This is most effective for stopping when players are running. When the first foot lands, the player should bend their knee to stop forward movement. The first foot to land is their pivot foot, if they have the ball.

Moving and Stopping

Jumping:	Players need to be able to jump off either foot and off two feet. And they must be able to do that standing still or on the run.
Change Direction:	Don't assume players can do this well. Teach them to push off the leg that is opposite to where they are going. They need to bend the knee and push hard.
Start Moving	Most children don't do this well. Players will tend to be left or right "footed" and will tend to always push of that foot. Many players take a step backwards to move forward!

Teach basic movement skills by giving players the chance to practice jumping and changing direction, through a range of fun activities.

Some of the best activities that you can use for improving fundamental movement skills are to adapt some simple games that kids play.

Fun Team Games to teach Fundamental Movement

Tag

Pick 3 or 4 players to be "it" and the rest of the players try to avoid being tagged. The "it" players have one ball and can only tag a player by touching them with the ball, while it is in the hands of the "it" player.

The "it" players pass them ball between themselves but cannot run with it. This emphasises pivoting, catching, and passing skills. When tagged a player can either move to the side or stand still. If they are standing still a team mate can "free" them by stepping between their legs.

Dribble Tag

In this game, each player that is "it" has a ball and must dribble it whilst they chase other players and try and tag them. They tag with their hand.

If you have enough balls, have every player dribble.

Guard the Castle

Have 3 or 4 players standing at half way - they are the guards. The other players start on the baseline (which is the sea) and have to get to the castle (the other baseline).

If a player is tagged by one of the guards, they must return to the "sea". You can have players dribble or introduce "gates", which limit the area that players can run through.

Three important things to look at when players move are:

- head position;
- which foot they push off; and
- bending their knees.

The position of the head is very important because if it moves away from "centre" it drastically affects the ability to move. Simply, the head has to move back to "centre" before they can change direction.

What is the correct footwork?

To move to your left, push off your right foot and step with your left foot. Many people don't do this!

Another common mistake is when starting to run forward - people often take a small step backwards (to push off) before moving forwards.

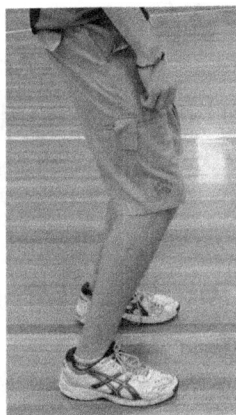

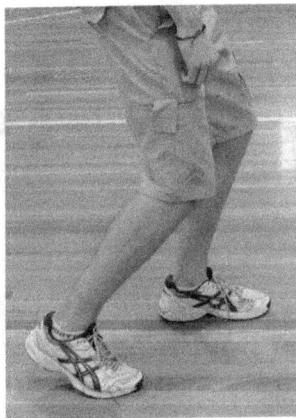

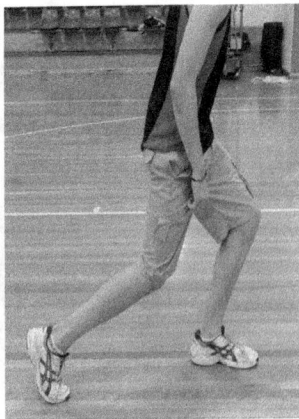

Sometimes, this may be because the person's feet are too far apart, their knees aren't bent or their weight is on their heels.. However, more commonly it is just poor technique.

Correcting it is a matter of practicing it correctly, although this is easier than it sounds because they will have a very ingrained habit in how they move. Using a foot ladder (describe later in the book can be very effective).

Research indicates that rather than trying to change an established habit, it is more effective if you instead teach them a new habit.

This can be as simple as giving the skill a new name (eg "sharp turns" instead of change direction), showing them the teaching points (knee bend, push off the foot opposite to the direction you want to move) and then practicing that new skill.

It seems that our brains are better wired for learning new skills than "unlearning" old ones. It is very important when they "revert" back to their old habit that you don't talk to them about what they have done (the "old way") and try to change it.

Instead, focus on the new skill and tell them what you want them to do - the new teaching points.

Every player needs to be able to "handle" the ball. Below are the key basics:

Passing and Catching	
Catching	Too often overlooked, catching is a skill and needs to be taught. Players need to have "soft" hands, allowing the ball to come to them and not grab at it. However, once caught, they need to have a strong grip on the ball! When teaching players to catch, the following tips are useful: • Have your fingers pointing up. Many players that don't catch well, have previously hurt their fingers when the ball hit them on the end of the fingers; • Keep your eyes open! Again, if they have hurt their fingers before, they may close their eyes or look away at the moment of catching. • Have a player stand with hands up and push the ball into their hands to practice. Gradually step backwards and pass the ball to them.

Passing and Catching

Chest Pass	A two handed pass. Start with both thumbs behind the ball, pointing at each other and the other fingers spread on the ball. 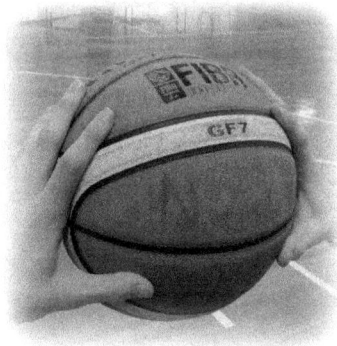
	Step forward as you pass and push both arms forward. Finish with straight arms, thumbs pointing to the ground and fingers pointing at your target. 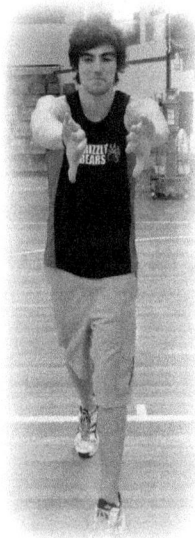

Passing and Catching

"Push pass"	A "push pass" is a one handed pass and players need to be able to throw it with both hands.
	Keep the passing hand behind the ball, and the other hand on the side to give a good grip. As shown below, this is the same grip on the ball as for shooting.

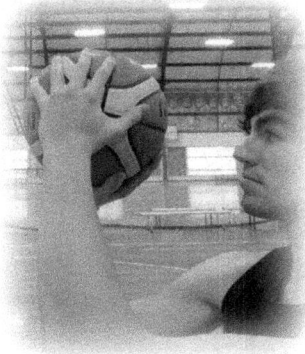 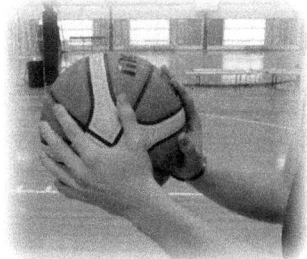

Shooting   Passing

Step toward the target as you pass and extend both arms. However, only the passing hand pushes the ball. The other arm extends to protect the ball from the defender.

Passing and Catching

Bounce Pass	Either a chest pass or a "push" pass can be used as a bounce pass. Simply, a bounce pass bounces on the floor before reaching the target. The ball should bounce up to the waist of the person receiving it.
Overhead Pass	Keep the ball above your head, but in front of your forehead (you should not lose sight of the ball). It takes a lot of strength to throw this pass over distance.

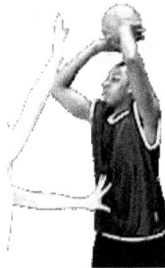

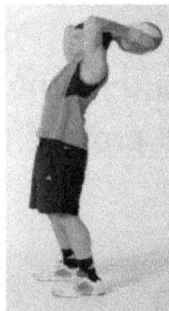

This allows a player to grab the ball from behind.

"Fake it to Make it"

A fake is only effective if someone believes it's real!

Simply, a pass fake must look like a pass! Use a fake to create a passing lane—"fake high, pass low" or "fake low, pass high.

A common mistake that players make is to make their fakes so fast that the defender doesn't have time to react or they (the offensive player) are not looking to see what reaction the defender makes.

Avoid boring repetitive drills

Passing is commonly taught by having players in pairs pass the ball back and forth to each other. This very quickly becomes boring. It is also quite unrealistic, because in a game, it is rare that a pass is made where:

- Both passer and catcher are unguarded;
- Both passer and catcher are standing still;
- Passer and catcher throw the ball repeatedly to each other.

This static form of "pairs passing" should not be used for very long. If you are using it, you should consider:

- Have players alternate the foot they step forward with as they pass the ball;
- Challenge players by seeing how many passes they can make in a set time;

- Use groups of 4, not 2, and have them moving to the next line after they pass. Also, have them leading for the ball (even if it is two steps in one direction and then back toward the ball);

- When practicing bounce passes, put a large coin on the floor. Players try to move the coin toward their partner by having the ball hit the coin.

Here is a contested version of "pairs passing" that is a good way to practice passing under pressure.

Groups of at least four, start on the baseline. First person dribbles to the foul line and jump stops. The second person runs behind them.

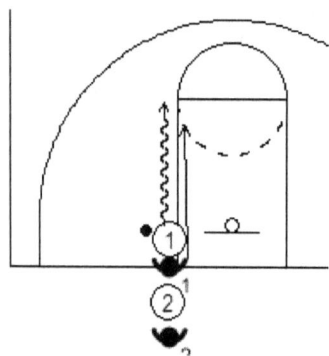

First person turns to face the baseline. They should look to see the defender (by putting chin to shoulder) and pivot to move away from the defender.

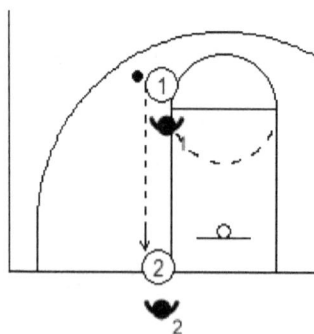

First person makes pass to the next person on the baseline. The defender tries to make the pass as hard as possible.

The best way to learn how to pass, and which pass to use, is to practice passing in "game like" activities.

Don't do all the thinking for the athlete - they will learn more from trying the wrong type of pass (and realising that it doesn't work) than from you stopping activities to tell them what type of pass to make.

If you want to talk about mistakes they made, ask open ended questions like "why was it hard to pass the ball to Jane" or "what did you see when you made the pass"?

Great Team Activities to Practice Passing

There are many games and activities that you can use to emphasise passing and developing the skills of being able to use a range of passes and knowing which pass to use.

Keeping's Off

Perhaps the simplest game is "keeping's off", where one team tries to make a certain number of passes (eg 100) without the other team gaining control of the ball.

There are a number of variations you can add:

- Each person on the team has to receive a minimum number of passes. This can emphasise the use of "screening" to help get a team mate open;
- Include an area on the court where a catch is worth double (eg centre circle).

V Lead Drill

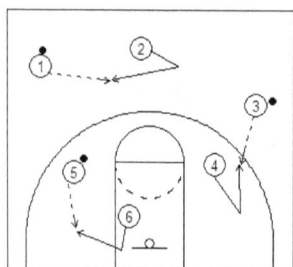

Pairs (or groups of 3) have one ball. The person who is going to catch the ball, takes 2 or 3 steps away and then cuts back toward the ball.

They should catch the ball "in the air" and then can alternate using a jump stop or stride stop.

4 Lanes Passing

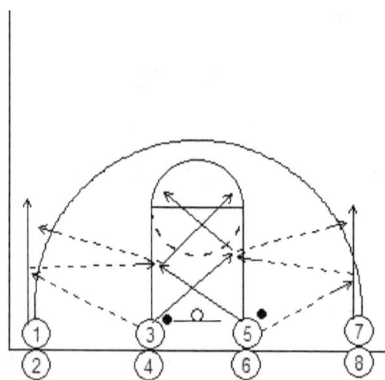

This is a very versatile drill and you can use many variations. You would usually do it full court, but could do it half court.

In the drill shown, there are four lines and the players in the middle two lines have a ball.

They pass the ball to the outside line and then cut toward the other line to receive a pass. They continue this full court and a shot is taken at the other end. It can be either one a lay-up or outside jump shot.

You can even have some defenders on the court to try to intercept passes!

Dribbling

All players must also be able to dribble the ball. The secret to dribbling is to push the ball, the harder you push it the more likely it will come back to your hand.

To have players realise this, get them to dribble with their fingers held straight—batting at the ball. They will quickly realise they do not have much control.

Then have them bend their fingers and let the ball bounce into their hands before pushing it down, bending at the wrist. They will quickly realise this gives them better control!

You also need to help them not to look at the ball when they dribble - instead they need to "see" with their fingers. However, remember to use positive language (tell them what to look at it) rather than just saying "don't look down".

What should they look at? Have them look at you, other players on the court, a spot on the wall - it really doesn't matter. One thing that can be effective is to have them pass the ball when their partner puts their hands up. This emphasises good catching technique as well as helping them develop their dribbling.

You can also use use activities where instructions are given by signals. This can be as simple as holding your hand up to show which hand they have to dribble with or pointing in the direction you want them to dribble.

Having them dribble when there is a lot of "traffic" on the court (ie lots of players on court at the same time) will help them to look up, otherwise they will run into other people!

Dribbling	
Crossover Dribble	Change hands by bouncing the ball in front from one hand to the other (by bouncing on the floor). The ball should stay below the knee. It is important to have your "catching" down and ready to receive the ball.
Hesitation Dribble	Also called a "stop/go move", this is where the dribbler looks like they going to stop, but then continues again. Stop your feet and keep knees bent. Dribble the ball slightly higher - coming up to the waist. Lift the shoulders and head slightly as well. Then push the ball forward and step forward to continue dribble. Make sure players don't put their hand underneath the ball as this is an illegal dribble.

Dribbling	
Retreat Dribble	It is often necessary to dribble backwards. Turn slightly sideways, but keep looking ahead. Dribble the ball near your back foot. Keep the other arm up to protect the ball. Move backwards at a slight angle and then be ready to dribble past your opponent.
Behind the back dribble	This is another way to change hands but uses your body to protect the ball. The key to doing this successfully is: • Don't dribble the ball in front of your body, to start the ball should be dribbling at your side; • Slide your dribbling hand so that it is behind the ball, rather than on top of it; • Push the ball forward, slap your bottom with your dribbling hand. The most common mistake is pushing the ball sideways, not in front (which makes it very hard to run forwards).

Dribbling

Onside Move (or Fake Crossover)	With this move, the player pretends to change direction. There are two different moves - let's assume you are dribbling right hand:
	• Push the ball toward the left hand side. Then roll your hand over the top of the ball (before it hits the floor) and push the ball back to the right. The ball hits the floor ONCE.
	• Bounce the ball on the floor toward your left. Move your right hand to the other side of the ball and dribble the ball back to your right. The ball hits the floor TWICE.
	The footwork is the same, small step to your left (left foot) and then push off your left foot and take big step to your right.
	It will also help "sell" the fake, if the player turns their shoulders slightly to their left, as they make the dribble move.

Dribbling	
Between the legs	This is used to change direction, or change hands and protects the ball with the body.
	Have one foot in front of the other. If dribbling right hand, have the left foot forward. Dribble the ball so that it hits the floor underneath your body - as it goes between your legs.
	Practice using a stride stop and then dribble between the legs.

Combined Dribble Moves

Players must be able to combine dribble moves. For example a fake crossover followed by a crossover. And remember, it's not a fake unless someone thinks it's real. Many players make fakes, but do not then take the time to see what reaction (if any) the defender has made. For example:

- If you fake a drive and the defender adjusts to guard it - make a crossover move and go the other way;

- If you fake a drive and the defender makes no reaction then drive in that direction!

There are other dribble moves and, most notably, we have not included the reverse pivot dribble. This can be a very effective way to protect the ball (as you turn your back to the defender) but particularly with young players, it often leads them into trouble as they lose sight of the defenders altogther.

Indeed, many coaches have a defensive rule that a reverse pivot dribble is automatically an opportunity to double team the dribbler.

The Golden Rule of Dribbling
Don't be fancy, be effective!
Too many players use lots of dribble moves but don't focus on what is important - beating their defender! A dribble move should either be used to protect the ball or as an attempt to get past the defender.

Players always attack the legs of their defender and step past them. Your hip should be lower than theirs.

Dribble moves often need to be accompanied with movement of the feet (a small step to make it look like you are changing direction) or movement of the upper body and shoulders. For example, when a player moves to their left, they will almost always turn their body left. Accordingly, a fake to go left should include turning shoulders to the left.

Finally, keep your head UP! For three reasons:

- To see open teammates (and pass them the ball);
- To see defenders that may be coming to help;
- To see your defender (so you can beat them!)

Great team activities to practice dribbling

A simple activity that particularly emphasises keeping your eyes up when dribbling is Dribble Chicken.

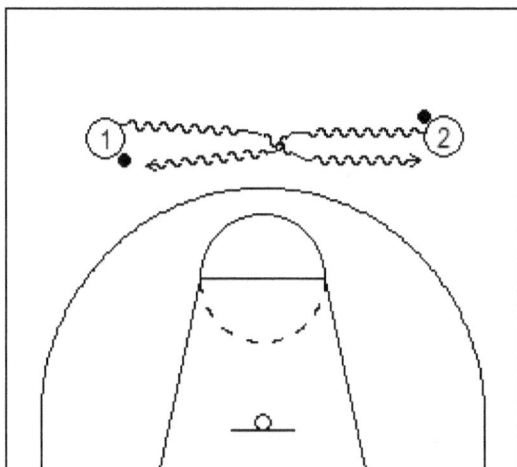

Two athletes (each with a ball) stand opposite each other. They must start dribbling with the same hand, which requires some communication.

They dribble straight at each other before making a dribble move (crossover, fake crossover etc). They should make the same move and should treat the other player as a defender - staying low as they make they make the move.

Add some "traffic" onto the court, which emphasises that athletes "looking up", by having groups do dribble chicken but in different directions:

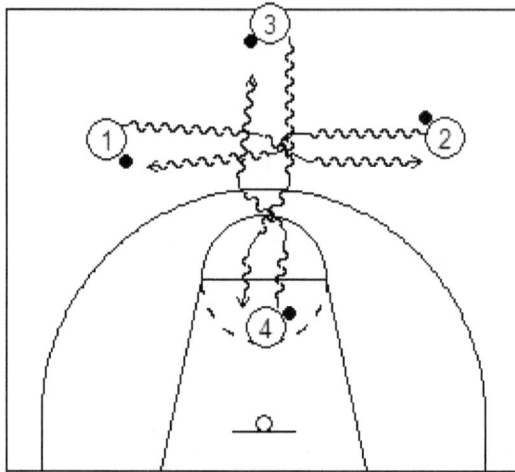

Here, when O_1 and O_2 get close to each other, they make their dribble move and then dribble past each other. O_3 and O_4 do the same thing. However, they must avoid contact with other players.

If O_3 is close to O_1, they should hesitate, retreat or stop their dribble and then accelerate to move into the gap.

This activity can be done in a half court with up to 16 athletes (8 pairs). It does get chaotic but it will certainly keep their heads up.

Team Dribble Knock Out

"Dribble Knock Out" is an activity commonly used by coaches where every player has a ball and they dribble in a set area of the court (half court, inside the 3pt line, within the key). Each player dribbles their own ball and tries to knock away the balls of other players.

Here is a team version of the same game:

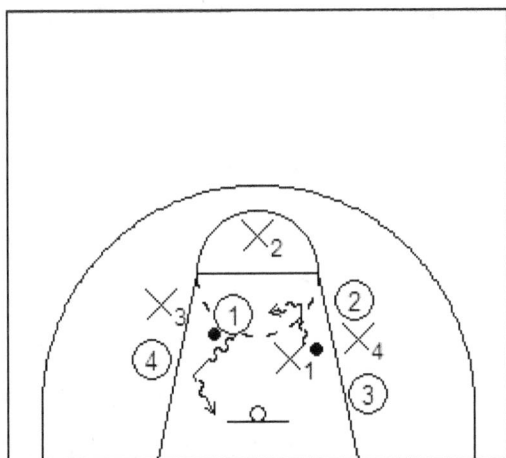

One person from each team has a ball and is in the key. Here we have shown two teams of 4, but the activity can be done with up to 4 teams.

The players in the key dribble their ball and try to knock the other person's ball away, while dribbling their own. If a player's ball is knocked out of the area, they step out, and a team mate replaces them.

Team Dribble Knock Out continued

The team to have all team members "knocked out" first losesl Not only can the people in the key knock the ball away but the players standing outside the key also try to knock balls away. They cannot step into the key but can move around if they wish.

The dribbler must be conscious not only of the players in the key but also who is behind them or outside the key.

Full Court Star Passing Drill

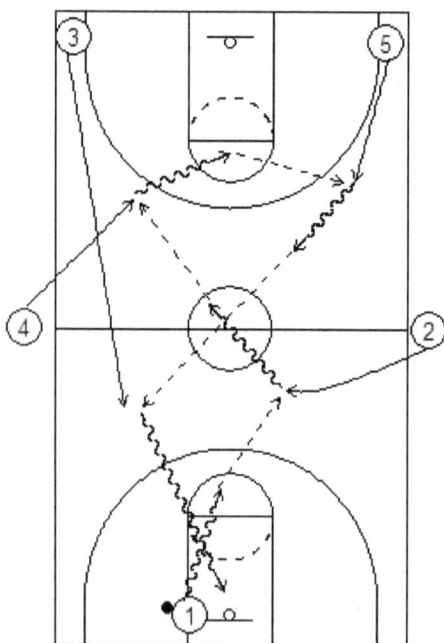

This drill practices passing on the to someone moving. After passing you join the line you passed to. Two or three dribbles at most:

- O_1 starts in the key and passes to O_2.
- O_2 passes to O_4
- O_4 passes to O_5 (O_3 starts to sprint at same time)
- O_5 passes to O_3 who shoots a lay-up. The next person in O_1's line rebounds the shot

Improving Footwork and Agility

> *Basketball requires quick feet. If you cannot move your feet, you cannot play basketball.*
>
> **Phil Jackson**

Equipment

To help improve the footwork and agility of you're athletes the following equipment may be useful:

- Foot ladder;
- Skipping Ropes;
- Cones.

Activities

Foot Ladder Activities

Using a foot ladder is a great way to improve agility and foot speed. If you don't have a ladder, you could simply mark a ladder with tape or chalk.

Foot ladders can be used anywhere and we describe just some of the different patterns that can be used.

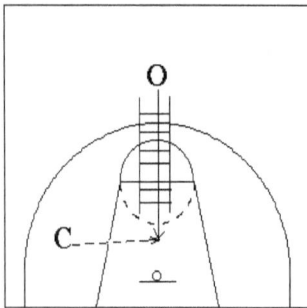

Set up the foot ladder near a basket and have athletes hold a ball, or receive a pass from the coach, before taking one step and shooting as they leave the ladder. Always alternate left and right handed shots.

When using the foot ladder athletes must:

- Be as quiet as possible (minimise feet hitting the floor);
- Keep their "nose behind their toes" - leaning forward will affect both balance and speed

Straight Run

Place one foot in each square of the ladder. Go through twice, alternating which foot takes the first step.

Two Foot Run

Run through the ladder with each foot stepping into each square. Alternate whether your first step is with the left or right.

"Two In, Two Out" - Front on run

Facing forward, place two feet in the first square and step outside the ladder. Natural running motion (right-left-right-left) should be used.

"Two In, Two Out" - Side on run

Stand on the side of the ladder and then step two feet into the ladder and two feet outside. Make sure you do it on both sides of the ladder to alternate which is the "lead" foot.

Diagonal

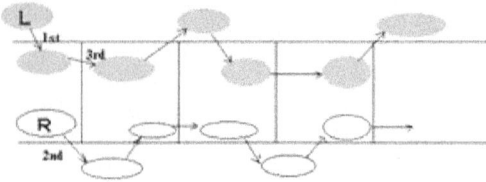

Start with one foot outside and one foot in the ladder. Step "In" (two feet in the square) -"Out" (other foot steps out) -"Up" (foot that is in moves forward to the next square). Practice doing backwards as well.

Hop

Hop through the ladder, landing in every second square. Have players reach up as if shooting a lay-up (if hopping on right foot, reach with left arm). To emphasise jumping up, have them also hop into every square.

"In Out" run

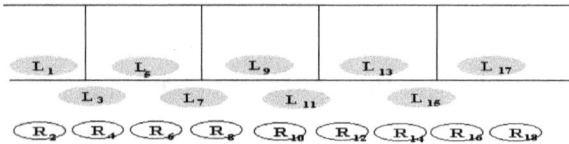

Run through the ladder. One foot remaining outside the ladder and the other foot stepping in and out of the ladder. Make sure players maintains "left-right" stepping..

"Crab Step"

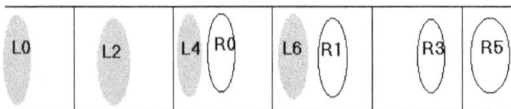

This is similar to defensive footwork. Start with both feet in the ladder, with one square empty between feet. Step with the "lead" foot, to make two squares between feet. Then bring back foot up, to return to one square empty. Do drill at least twice, facing opposite ways.

Activities

Run the Lines

Athletes start in the corner and must run along the lines. Every time they come to a new line they must change direction. Make sure they push off the "outside foot" (ie if they are moving to their left, they push of their right foot).

Variations

- Have players dribble while running along the lines

- "Pac Man" - 3 players start from a different point and they must try to tag the other players. Any player that steps off the line is out.

Touch the Ball

Stand behind the ball, which rests on the ground. Jump in the air and land with right foot on the floor and left foot on the ball. Jump again and switch feet. The foot landing on the ball must land lightly, so the ball doesn't move.

This drill helps develop controlled placement of the feet.

Scissor Jumps

Athletes stand on baseline, with one foot behind baseline and one foot in front of baseline. On command, athlete switches feet either once, twice or three times. Continue drill for 30 seconds.

Activities

Side Jumps

Athlete starts in a defensive stance, with feet comfortably apart. Jump off one foot and land on the other foot. Then jump back the other direction. Athletes should look to jump further and further, but always land balanced. Goal is to be able to jump the length of the foul line.

Ball Jumps

Athlete jumps continuously over the ball - either side to side or forward-backwards. See how many jumps they can do in 30 seconds.

Change direction sprints

Athlete starts on the baseline (up to 3 athletes at a time). They sprint in the direction that the coach points. When the coach claps, they sprint to the end of the court and the next athlete/group starts.

Athletes should concentrate on pushing off the "outside" foot (ie moving to the right, push off the left foot) and staying low and balanced.

Have them sprint forwards and backwards as well as left and right. As a variation, have the athletes dribble.

Activities

Skipping Rope

Skipping improves footwork, as it emphasises quick contact with the floor. It will also help rebounding, helping the athlete "jump, land, jump again". Challenge your athletes with the following:

Basic Jumps

Turn the rope in circles using your wrist and hands. Jump over the rope as it hits the floor, landing on two feet. Practice with the rope circling in a clockwise direction (start with it behind your feet) and anti-clockwise (start with it in front of feet)

Double / Triple Jumps

Once athlete can do the basic jump, have them turn the rope faster so that it passes underneath them two or three times in one jump. They can also jump higher.

Running Step

Start with rope in front of your feet and raise knees high in a running motion. The other foot lifts off the ground sufficient for the rope to pass underneath.

Hop

Athlete hops on one foot to jump over the rope.

Moving Scissor

Start with one foot in front of the other. Jump the rope, switching feet.

Activities

Skipping Rope (continued)

Arms Cross

Athlete stands with feet together and the rope behind their heels. Bring the rope above the head, crossing arms at the elbow. On the next turn they "un-cross" their arms.

Legs Cross

Athlete jumps the rope and lands with feet apart. Next time, they land with feet crossed, right foot in front. Next jump, land feet apart and lastly (in the pattern) land with feet crossed, left foot in front.

Box Jump

Athlete jumps with two feet. First, they jump forward. Next jump is to the left, then backwards and then to the right (which should bring them to their starting position).

This activity can be done while hopping as well.

Remember: when turning the rope the athlete should try not to be moving their whole arm and instead use their wrists.

Improving Reaction and Anticipation

> *If I wait to see what you do and then react, I'll be slower than you. I want to anticipate what you will do, act first and then you have to react to me!*
>
> **Michael Haynes**

Improving Reaction and Anticipation

Good athletes are able to react quickly to what is happening on the court. Great athletes are able to anticipate what will happen and act before it does!

Reaction and anticipation can be improved three ways:

- Giving your athletes cues / tips on what to look at to anticipate what will happen;
- Letting your athletes develop confidence in their ability to anticipate - don't constantly stop activities;
- Practice reacting to different situations.

Importantly, anticipation is different to guessing. Anticipation involves "reading" both "the play" and individual athletes.

1/2 Turn Calls

1 athlete stands in a defensive stance (in black below), facing a coach and two other athletes stand to each side. The coach passes to an athlete on the side, who passes it to the athlete in the middle. Before catching the ball the athlete in the middle must jump to face the passer. After catching it, they jump back to face the coach and then pass to the coach.

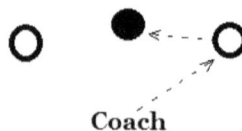

O   ● <- - - O

Coach

1/2 Turn Calls (continued)

Tips to anticipate the coach's pass

The athlete should "read" where the coach is going to pass the ball, and then may start to turn in that direction. If the coach has the ball on their right hand side, they are more likely to pass to their right.

Similarly, if the coach has turned their chest toward a player (which you can often identify by the turn of their shoulders), they are likely to pass to that player, even if they are looking the other way!

Blind Catch

An athlete stands in front of the coach, facing away from the coach. The Coach calls "left" or "right" and passes the ball at the same time. The athlete must turn in that direction and catch the pass.

The athlete should get vision of the ball as quickly as possible, by turning their head—putting the chin on their shoulder.

Blind Turn Calls

Athlete stands an arm's length away from the coach, facing away from the coach. The coach holds the ball at shoulder height and drops the ball as they call "left" or "right". The player turns in that direction and must catch the ball before it touches the ground. Again, "chin to shoulder" to get vision!

Body Touch

Athlete stands in a defensive stance, facing the coach, and holding the ball at their chin. Coach calls out "Ears", "Shoulders", "Stomach", "Backside" or "Knees".

The athlete lets the ball go, touches that part of their body, and then catches the ball before it hits the ground. The athlete must stay in defensive stance.

The coach may assign a number to each body part.

Line Touch

Athletes stand on the "split line" and on the coach's command run to touch a side line and then sprint back to their starting position. Initially, coach would call "left" or "right".

To develop ability to anticipate, the coach has a ball and the players sprint when the coach dribbles in one direction. The coach may fake before dribbling.

Tips to "Reading" the Coach

As with passers, if the coach has their chest turned in a direction, that is the direction they are likely to move. The lower they are holding the ball, the more likely they are going to actually dribble.

As the players anticipate the direction the coach may move, they take a step in that direction, always moving both their feet.

Intercept the pass

Coach has the ball at the top of the key, with two players on each wing. Defender starts on the foul line and tries to intercept the coach's pass.

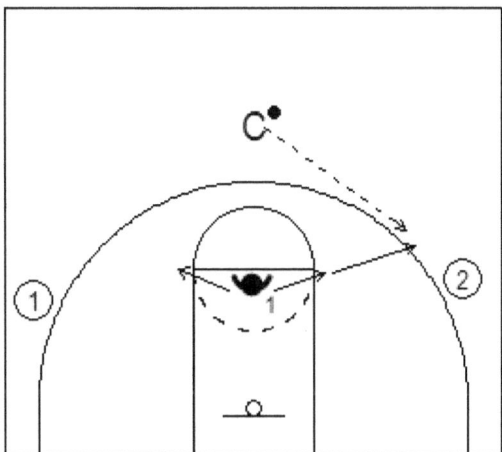

The defender should move to the side of the key as they anticipate where the coach may pass. It is easiest to intercept the pass close to the offensive player as it gives longer to get to the pass and if they miss the intercept, they are closer to them.

Triangle Pass Hedging Drill

This activity has two defenders and three offensive players. One of the defensive players must always guard the ball while the other defender "guards 2" - trying to intercept a pass.

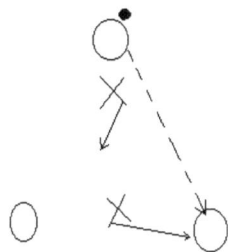

In addition to "reading" the passer, the intercepting defender should "read" where their team mate is. If the team mate is on the left hand side, the passer will probably pass right handed. If the teammate has a hand up, the pass will probably be a bounce pass.

Developing Basketball Fitness

The main physical traits you need to play basketball are endurance, agility and strength. I would start with a program that increases stamina because once fatigue sets in it will negatively affect the way you play.

Ten G

"Plyo" Rebounds

One athlete stands on a chair holding a ball so it is out of reach of their partner. The partner jumps to touch the ball with their right hand, lands and immediately jumps to touch it with their left hand.

After they have touched the ball 10 times (5 left, 5 right), they jump and grab it with both hands.

Alternatively, have athlete run and jump off one foot to touch the ball—this practices their lay-ups!

Sprint Dribbles

Have players start on the baseline with a basketball. They should be dribbling while standing still.

On your command, they dribble past the foul line and then retreat dribble back to the baseline. They change hands and dribble out again.

This continues for 30 seconds, and then they stand on the baseline, dribbling on the sport, for 10-15 seconds. This is their rest period.

Continue the activity for 3 or 4 minutes.

You can also do this activity from the "wing" position, and have them dribble into the key.

O'Brien's Catch & Shoot Drill

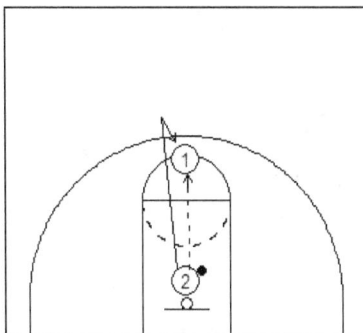

O_2 passes to O_1 who shoots. O_2 runs out to pressure the shot and then goes out the 3pt line. O_1 rebounds their shot and then passes to O_2.

The defender should run past the shooter, past their shooting arm. If they run across the player they are more likely to foul.

Continue until one player makes 10 shots, however if a rebound touches the floor they lose a shot!

Players should "catch and shoot" if they can, however if the defender is close, they should fake a shot and then take one dribble. The defender runs past.

If a defender tips the shot, they earn an extra point and they also earn a point if they cause the offensive player to fake a shot.

O'Brien's Lay-up Drill

O_1 catches pass from coach and then does a lay-up. The other coaches rebounds the ball, passes it to the top of the key and O_1 then leads to receive pass at the wing.

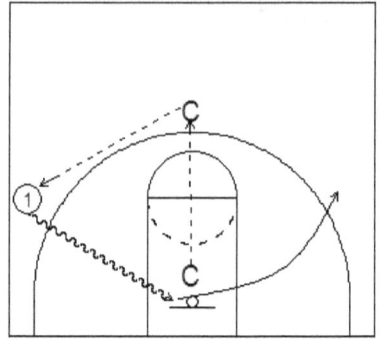

O_1 should only take one dribble for each lay-up and can alternate whether they forward pivot (to face the basket) or reverse pivot (straight into lay-up). On a forward pivot they may "rip through" and drive baseline or drive middle.

O_1 should shoot at least 13 shots in one minute.

Full Court Jump Shots

Athletes dribble to the foul line and take a jump shot - this is not a free throw and there should be no pause. They rebound the shot. If the shot missed, they shoot lay-ups until they get a score.

Athlete then dribbles to the other end for a shot from the foul line. If they made their first shot, they dribble sprint to half way and then can jog to the free throw line. If they missed the first shot, they dribble sprint the whole way.

Continue until they have made a certain number of shots (eg 16) or for a certain time (3-5 mins).

Close Out Conditioner

X_1 starts with the ball and passes to O_1. X_1 then "closes out" toward O_1. Sprinting toward them but stopping in front ready to defend.

As they get close to the player with the ball they should start to take small steps as they slow down and bring both hands up in front of them, which will help to keep their head and weight back.

X_1 "mirrors" the ball keeping their hands in front of the ball as O_1 pivots to protect the ball. If O_1 moves their feet, X_1 must move BOTH feet. After 5 secs X_1 jogs back to sideline and receives a pass from O_1 before starting again.

Alternatively, (shown by X_2) the defender uses "defensive slide" back to their position.

Full Court Shooting

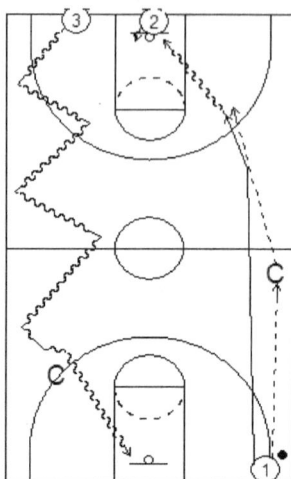

The athlete in this drill shoots three times and up to three players can be on court at the same time.

First, O_1 passes to the coach and then sprints full court. The Coach throws the ball ahead of them, and they catch and shoot a lay-up. They rebound their own shot.

Secondly, O_2 shoots a reverse lay-up. Starting on the baseline and taking two steps. If they are shooting right hand, their first step is with the right foot. Players should keep the ball at chest height.

Lastly, O_3 dribbles full court, changing direction with different dribble moves before taking a lay-up or jump shot.

Full Court Lay-ups

Athletes dribble full court and shoot lay-ups for 1 minute. They should aim for no more than 4 dribbles to move down the court.

Players should use a "speed dribble", which bounces the ball directly in front of them. They dribble it with one hand and then the other which mimics natural running action.

They player also alternates left and right handed shots. Aim is to make 10 shots in 1 minute.

3 Point Conditioner

Athlete takes 3pt shots with a coach rebounding. They cannot take shots from consecutive spots so must relocate after each shot. Target is to make 50 in 5½ minutes.

Can also do 2pt shots, with athlete stepping outside the 3pt line after each shot and then stepping inside to "catch and shoot" or catching the ball at the 3pt line, shot fake and take one dribble.

10 second drill

Athlete starts on the foul line, facing the coach who is at the basket. Coach throws the ball anywhere and starts to count 10 secs (loudly). Athlete retrieves the ball, scores and returns to the foul line.

The athlete "rests" until the coach counts reaches 10, and then the drill starts again. Coach can dictate the shot that the athlete must make.

Continue drill for 3-5mins, with coach varying whether they throw the ball short or long.

Team Pursuit

Have teams of four start on opposite sides of the court. They sprint around the court (say 10 times) in a race. If one team overtakes the other team they automatically win.

They must run in "single file" and the player at the back must sprint to the front. Once they get to the front they call the next person to sprint to the front.

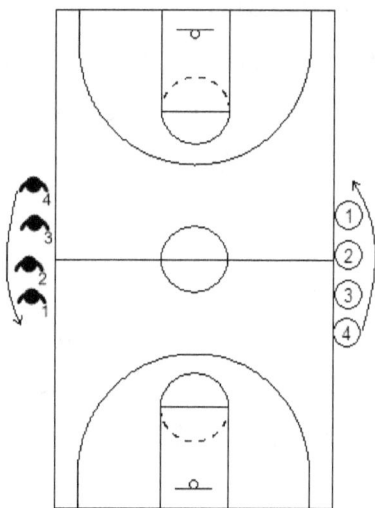

"Swish Shot" Drill

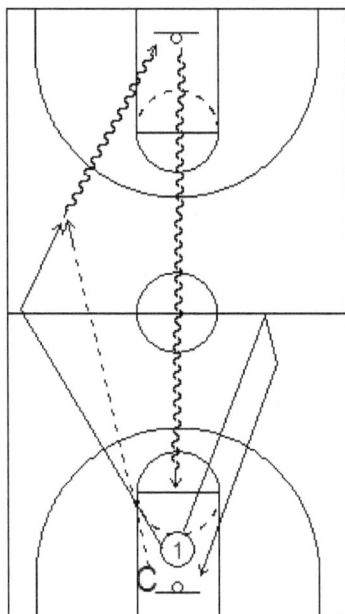

O_1 stands 1 or 2 steps in front of basket, taking shots. With experienced players you can even do this at the foul line

If the shot "swishes" (goes in, without hitting the ring or backboard) O_1 takes another.

If the shot went in, but hit the ring/backboard, O_1 sprints to half way and back.

If the shot misses, O_1 sprints to half way (wide) turns their head (chin to shoulder) to see and receive coach's pass before shooting lay-up. They then dribble back to take next shot.

Defend and Shoot Drill

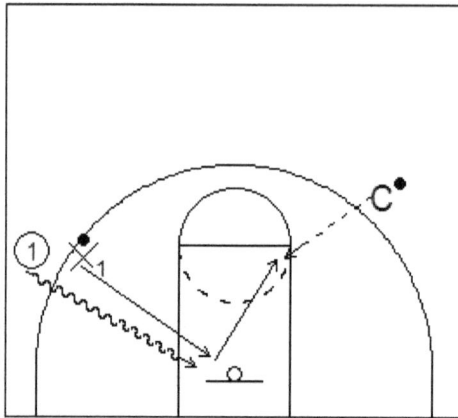

X_1 hands the ball to O_1 and then guards them 1v1. O_1 tries to get a lay-up, although you could simply make it that they try to get into the key.

After O_1 has scored or X_1 has secured the ball, X_1 passes to the Coach and then cuts to the foul line to receive a pass and shoot. X_1 rebounds their shot, passes to O_1 and starts again. Continue for 1 - 2mins.

You can make the activity competitive by awarding the defender a point if the offensive player doesn't score and also awarding them a point if they make their shot.

Munns Combo Drill

X_1 starts with the ball, hands it to O_1 and then defends O_1 who drives to the basket.

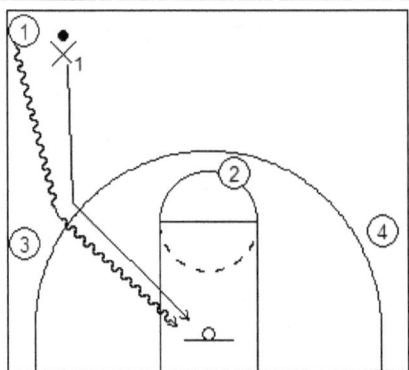

Once X_1 gets the ball (steal, rebound or O_1 scores), X_1 passes to the coach and moves to guard O_2 who tries to catch and shoot. X_1 must "box out" and if O_2 rebounds they play 1v1 until X_1 secures the ball.

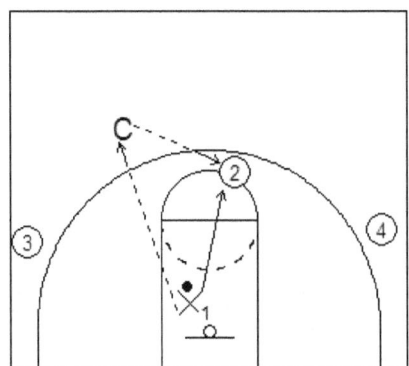

Once X_1 gets the ball they pass to the coach and then deny O_3 the ball. If O_3 gets the ball they play 1v1 until X_1 gets the ball.

If X_1 is able to deny O_3 getting the ball for 5 seconds they are given the ball.

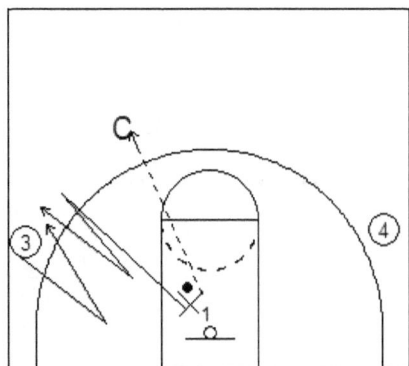

Munns Combo Drill (continued)

Once X_1 gets the ball in the 1v1 contest with O_3, they throw the ball to the coach and then move to guard O_4.
The coach may pass to O_4 on the wing, or O_4 may cut. They play 1v1.

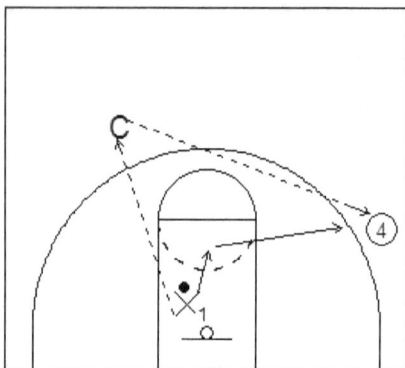

X_1 must hussle throughout the drill, as there is no break between the four parts. Where an offensive player scores, X_1 just catches the ball out of the net, step out of bounds and passes it back to the coach.

The rotation for the drill is:
   O_1 is the next defender
   X_1 moves to O_2
   O_2 moves to O_3
   O_3 moves to O_4
   O_4 moves to O_1

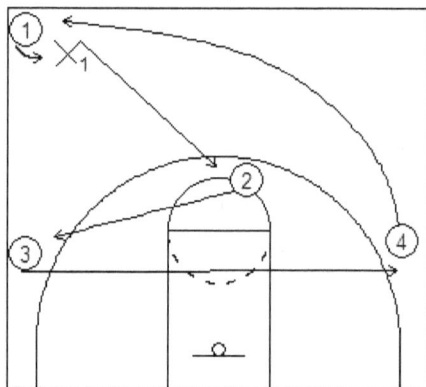

Learning to Control the Ball

> *We are all doing things that he [Pete Maravich] did first.*
>
> **Steve Nash**

Developing "Handles"

Regardless of what position they play, good players are able to control the ball. The ball must feel as though it is an extension of their hand.

For best control the ball should touch the fingers and the "balls" of the fingers (where the fingers joins the hand) but should not touch the palm of the hand.

Athletes should keep their hands "soft", so that all of their fingers touch the ball. They should let their fingers "see" the ball, using touch.

Another tip for developing good control of the ball is to use your "off hand" as much as possible. For example, if you are right handed, start to brush your teeth, open doors, put vegemite on your toast and operate the TV remote control with your left hand.

When doing the following activities, athletes should lose control of the ball sometimes - if they don't they are only doing what they already can do!

Pendulum

Hold the ball at your waist in both hands. Swing the ball in one hand up to shoulder height and then back down to your waist. Change hands and swing to the other side.

Wrap Arounds

Rotate the ball around your head, then waist, then knees and then ankles. Then work your way back up your body. Keep body still (particularly the head) and move the ball as quickly as possible.

Another version is to pass the ball around one leg, then both legs and then the other leg. Finally, a figure 8 around both legs, going in both clockwise and anti-clockwise direction.

Ball Drop

Hold the ball behind your head. Let the ball go and clap your hands in front of your body. Catch the ball (behind your back) before it hits the floor.

To increase difficulty, do more claps or drop the ball from lower.

Quick Hands

Hold the ball in both hands at knee height (either with both hands in front of your knees or one hand in front and the other behind).

Let go of the ball, switch hands and catch the ball before it hits the ground. If both hands were in front of your knee, catch the ball with both hands behind.

Under / Over

Hold the ball in both hands behind your body. Have your legs shoulder width apart. Bounce the ball through your legs and catch it with both hands in front of your hands. This is "under".

Throw the ball up in the air and catch it behind your back. This is "over". The key to this is to stand underneath the ball while it is in the air, watching it the whole time. As the ball drops, and almost hits your head, take a step forward and catch the ball. Keep your back straight.

Can alternate by starting with the ball in front, bouncing it under to the back and then throwing it over above the head.

Spider Dribble

Start with the ball in front of your body, legs apart. Have both hands in front of your body.

Bounce the ball with your right hand and then move your right hand behind your knees. Next bounce is with your left hand (in front of your knee) and then you move your left hand behind your knees.

Then bounce right hand (from behind), left hand (from behind), right hand (from in front), left hand (from in front) etc.

Weave Walk

As you walk, pass the ball between your legs. Walk in a crouched stance. Repeat walking backwards.

Wall Dribble

Stand 1m from the wall, facing the wall. Begin dribbling the ball against the wall, from about 15cm away from the wall. Dribble up and down the wall and then change hands.

Bridge

Kneel down on one knee, dribble the ball continuously under the bent knee. Add dribbling around the body or around their leg.

1 Ball Stationary Dribbling Athletes executing the following called by the coach.	
Front Continuously change hands dribbling in front of the body.	*Back* Continuously change hands dribbling behind the body.
Left/Right Hard Dribble the ball as hard as possible	*Left/Right* Dribble the ball in a "V" at the side of the body. The hand moves from the front to the back of the ball

1 Ball Stationary Dribbling (continued)
Athletes executing the following called by the coach.

Left/Right Round	*Left/Right Onside*
With one hand dribble the ball around the leg. Use 3-4 dribbles.	While dribbling take a small step with the opposite foot and an onside dribble.
Left/Right Front V	*Left/Right Hesitation*
Dribble with one hand in front of the body in a "V". The hand changes position to push the ball left and then right.	Dribble the ball low a hard. Then allow one dribble to rise higher, and then low again.
Spin Dribble	*Around the World*
Take three dribbles, jump stop and reverse pivot (90°). Step with the same foot as you are dribbling.	Dribble the ball 3 times with one hand and then change hands with a behind the back dribble.
Pull the ball back so that it bounces near the foot you have stepped with.	3 more dribbles on the spot and then change hands again with a crossover dribble.
Forward pivot and then take another 3 dribbles.	Change direction!

2 Ball Stationary Dribbling
Athletes executing the following called by the coach.

Front Dribble each ball once on the spot and then change hands.	*Side* Dribble each ball in a "V" at the side of the body.
Side Alternate Same as for the Side dribble, except as one hand is at the front of the body the other is at the back.	*Round* Dribble with right hand around right leg, then left hand around left leg. Do not change hands.
Behind and In Front Dribble 3 times on the spot and then change hands - one ball with a crossover in front of the body, the other with a behind the back dribble.	*Hesitate* Dribble the balls low and hard three times, then let one dribble rise higher.

Onside
Do onside dribbles with both balls. They should almost touch in the middle and should finish an arm's length distance from the body.

Bongo Drums Dribble

Have the athlete dribble three balls at the one time. Hard dribble two balls for 2 or 3 dribbles, then change both hands to a different ball (one ball will be continuously dribbled, but with alternating hands).

As the athlete develops confidence, have them dribble 4 balls.

Circle Dribble

Dribble stays in the jump ball circle with 1 or 2 defenders outside the circle. The defenders cannot step into the circle, but try to knock the ball away. The dribbler uses a variety of dribble moves as they move forward and backwards.

3 Dribble Change

O_1 starts at half way and dribbles toward the basket. They make 3 changes of direction with different moves.

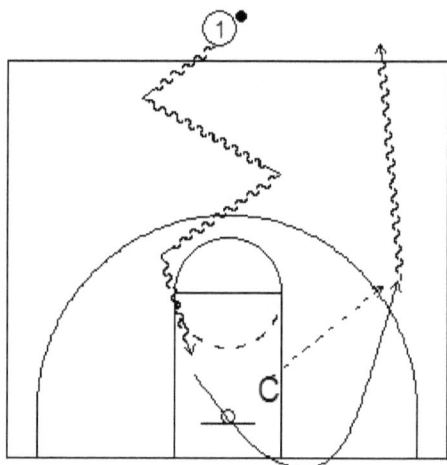

The coach calls to "shoot" or "lay-up" and the coach rebounds the ball.

After shooting, O_1 touches the baseline and sprints toward half way, receiving a pass from the coach and dribbling to half way.

Dribble Weaves

O_1 starts at half way and dribbles through the cones, using different moves to change direction.

They then do a lay-up (taking one dribble from 3pt line) and rebound their shot. They dribble to the 3pt line, change direction and dribbles to half way.

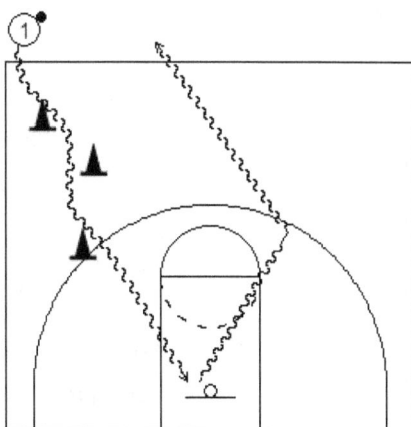

Foul line Dribble Sprint

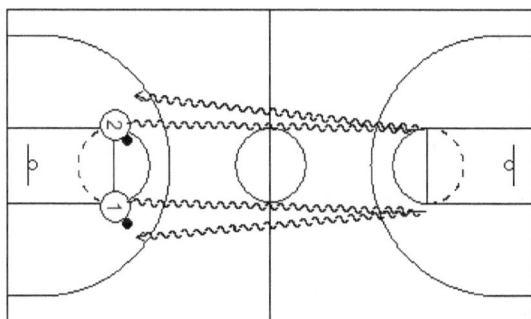

O_1 and O_2 start at foul line and dribble sprint to the other foul line and back. They should push the ball directly in front of them and dribble with alternating hands (which is natural running movement). Aim to do 14 to 15 in one minute.

Up and Backs

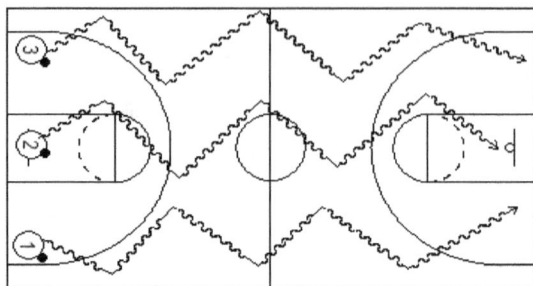

O_1, O_2 and O_3 dribble full court making 5 or 6 dribble moves. The should accelerate after making each moving, "beating" a defender. Alternatively, have athletes dribbling with two balls or add a defender. With a defender, do not allow them to touch the ball—emphasise getting their body in front and forcing the dribbler to change direction.

Gauntlet Drill

O_1 has to dribble past each defender. Defenders are not allowed to touch the ball - they must concentrate on getting good position.

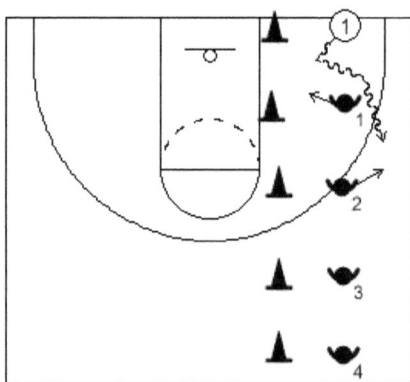

O_1 is not allowed to dribble out of the "corridor". The defenders guard the area near their "cone", and once beaten do not chase. O_1 may need to dribble backwards at times to get past!

2 Ball Shooting Drill

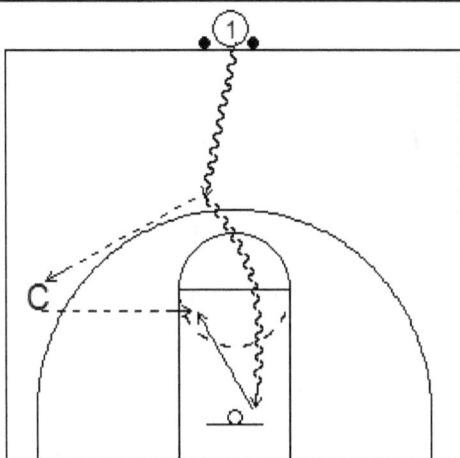

O_1 dribbles two balls from half way. At the 3pt line, they jump stop and pass to the coach with the hand closest to the coach. They keep dribbling the other ball while making this pass.

After passing, O_1 drives hard for a lay-up and then cuts back to the elbow to receive a pass from the coach for a jump shot. The coach changes sides while O_1 dribbles both balls back to half way.

Continue the drill until O_1 makes 10 jump shots - they lose 1pt for any missed lay-up.

2 Ball Passing Drill

Athlete is stationary, dribbling two balls. They pass one ball to the coach or a partner, while dribbling the other ball. The coach then passes the ball back - using a bounce pass initially as it is easier to catch.

As the athlete gets better, have them dribble one ball around their leg while passing the other. Or, have two athletes facing each other, both passing a ball with the same hand.

Chill Drill

O_1 dribbles around the court, making the following dribble moves:

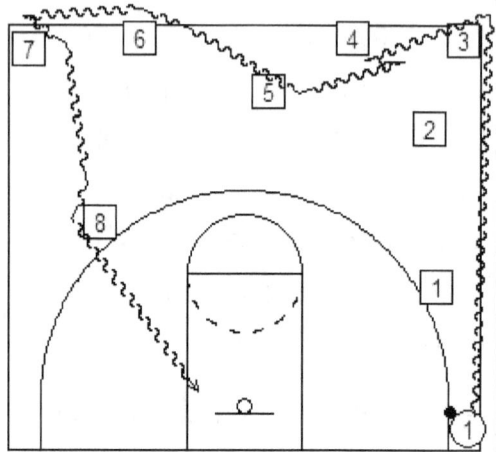

1. Onside Dribble (no change of hands)
2. Fake Crossover (no change of hands)
3. Reverse pivot (after jump stop)
4. Retreat Dribble (no change of hands)
5. Cross Over dribble
6. Between the legs and behind the back combination (change hands twice, so end up with no change!)
7. Behind the back (change hands)
8. Stutter step and cross over (change hands)

After the last move, the dribble hard to the basket for a lay-up, with one dribble from the 3pt line.

O_1 starts dribbling with their "outside hand" (closest to the sideline) - their right hand in the diagram. The drill should be done from both corners.

The Last Word

> *I think you want to try every sport possible, just to experience life.*
>
> **Jose Conseco**

The Last Word

When coaching, and particularly when coaching kids, keep perspective on why they are playing - mostly because it is fun and they do it with friends.

Some people say that winning is unimportant and shouldn't be a focus. I disagree. Winning, and losing, are important lessons to learn and apply as much in life as in sport.

What coaches must avoid is exclusively coaching to "win" - for example only playing their "better players" to try and win every game. Winning is not that important and every kid on the team should have the opportunity to participate.

What the coach must attempt to provide in every game, and at every training, is success! This is not necessarily winning. Learning how to perform a cross over dribble is success. Then doing that in a game and getting past a defender is another success.

I think all coaches should embrace the philosophy in a sign that I saw at a swimming school:

Dear Mum and Dad. Do not judge me on whether I win or lose my race. Judge me on what I can do now that I couldn't do when I first started.

www.ingramcontent.com/pod-product-compliance
Lightning Source LLC
LaVergne TN
LVHW021543080426
835509LV00019B/2805